Belly Fat Burner Diet

Quick and Delicious Recipes to Flatten Your Belly
and Keep You Fit For Life

Disclaimer and Terms of Use:

Effort has been made to ensure that the information in this book is accurate and complete, however, the author and the publisher do not warrant the accuracy of the information, text and graphics contained within the book due to the rapidly changing nature of science, research, known and unknown facts and internet. The Author and the publisher do not hold any responsibility for errors, omissions or contrary interpretation of the subject matter herein. This book is presented solely for motivational and informational purposes only.

Table of Contents

Introduction: 5

Belly Fat Burning Recipes 7

Tomato Basil Egg White Omelet............................ 8

Low-Fat Whole-Wheat Pancakes......................... 11

Strawberry Kale Green Smoothie 13

Spinach and Mushroom Egg Cups 15

Mixed Veggie Egg White Omelet......................... 17

Avocado Walnut Smoothie 19

Carrot and Ginger Soup 21

Creamy Chicken Apple Salad 23

Easy Tomato Basil Soup...................................... 25

Mediterranean Chopped Salad 27

Chicken and Vegetable Stew 29

Dairy-Free Tuna Salad... 31

Butternut Squash Soup with Curry 33

Simple Chicken Piccata 35

Grilled Balsamic Salmon Fillets........................... 37

Turkey Meatloaf 39

Slow Cooker Chicken Cacciatore 41

Almond-Crusted Baked Haddock........................ 43

Herbed Turkey Burgers....................................... 45

Baked Coconut Cod 47

Chia Seed Pudding with Berries................................... 49

Honey Poached Pears 51

Whole-Wheat Vanilla Cupcakes 53

Walnut-Stuffed Baked Apples 55

Cinnamon and Honey Baked Bananas.......................... 57

Conclusion 59

Introduction:

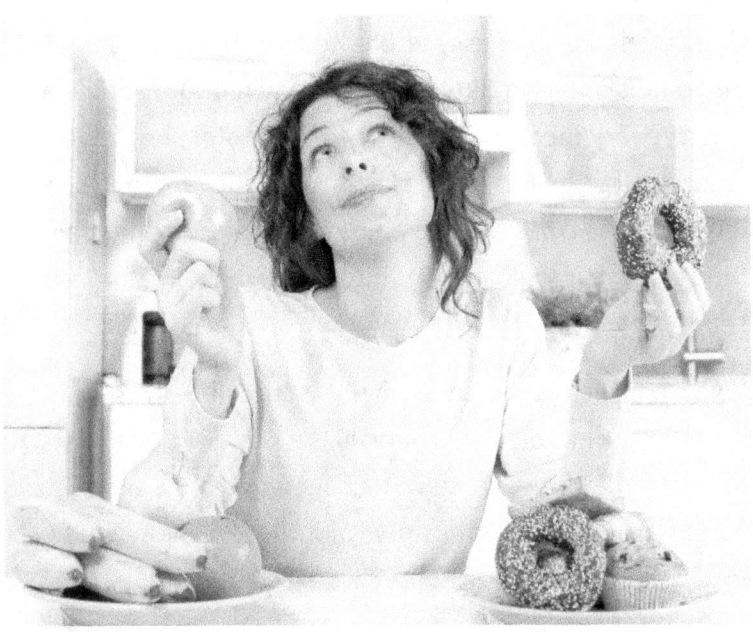

Are you carrying around a little extra weight – especially in the stomach area? Belly fat can be very stubborn and hard to get rid of but it is possible if you have the right tools at your disposal. The key to losing your stubborn belly fat is to make adjustments to your diet in terms of what you eat and how much you eat. You do not have to starve yourself in order to follow the belly fat burner diet. All you have to do is eat small 400-calorie meals four times a day (every four hours) and focus on healthy, wholesome foods.

When you switch to the belly fat burner diet you will need to reduce your consumption of processed foods and refined sugars. You should also avoid starchy foods like pasta and white bread. Try to drink plenty of water each day and do not add extra salt to your food. Avoid foods that can make you gassy or bloated like broccoli, onions, and beans and try to get some healthy monounsaturated fats at every meal. The majority of your diet should be composed of healthy fats, fresh fruits and vegetables, and whole grains. You can also enjoy fat-free or low-fat dairy in moderation as well as egg whites, lean protein, nuts, and seeds.

If you are ready to kiss your belly fat goodbye with the belly fat burner diet, this book is the perfect place to start. In this book you will receive a collection of 25 delicious recipes for the belly fat burner diet that will help you to lose that stubborn belly fat – fast.

Belly Fat Burning Recipes

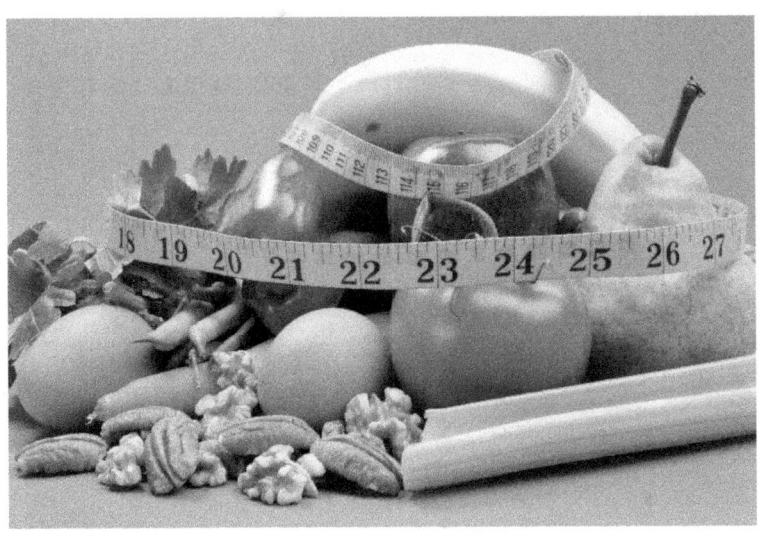

Recipes Included in this Book:

Tomato Basil Egg White Omelet

Mixed Veggie Egg White Omelet

Low-Fat Whole-Wheat Pancakes

Avocado Walnut Smoothie

Strawberry Kale Green Smoothie

Carrot and Ginger Soup

Spinach and Mushroom Egg Cups

Creamy Chicken Apple Salad

Easy Tomato Basil Soup

Mediterranean Chopped Salad

Chicken and Vegetable Stew

Dairy-Free Tuna Salad

Butternut Squash Soup with Curry

Simple Chicken Piccata

Grilled Balsamic Salmon Fillets

Turkey Meatloaf

Slow Cooker Chicken Cacciatore

Almond-Crusted Baked Haddock

Herbed Turkey Burgers

Baked Coconut Cod

Chia Seed Pudding with Berries

Honey Poached Pears

Whole-Wheat Vanilla Cupcakes

Walnut-Stuffed Baked Apples

Cinnamon and Honey Baked Bananas

Tomato Basil Egg White Omelet

Servings: 1

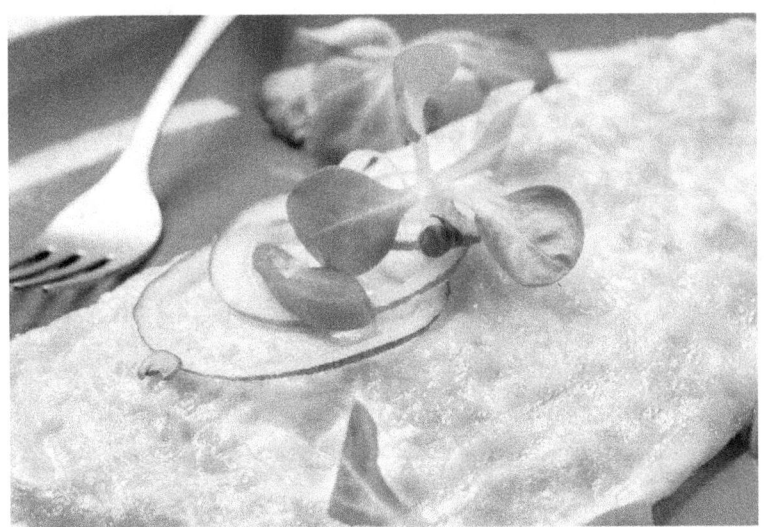

Ingredients:

- 2 teaspoons olive oil, divided
- 1 medium Roma tomato, chopped
- 1 clove minced garlic
- 3 large egg whites, beaten
- 1 tablespoon fresh chopped chives
- Pinch fresh ground pepper
- 1 tablespoon fresh chopped basil

Instructions:

1. Heat 1 teaspoon oil in a small skillet over medium heat.
2. Add the tomato and garlic and cook for 3 minutes.
3. Spoon the tomato mixture into a bowl and reheat the skillet with the rest of the oil.

4. Beat together the egg whites, chives and fresh pepper.
5. Pour the eggs into the skillet and cook for 1 minute then stir gently.
6. Cook the eggs for another 2 to 3 minutes until almost set.
7. Spoon the tomato mixture over half the omelet and sprinkle with basil.
8. Fold the omelet over and cook for 1 minute or until the eggs are set.

Low-Fat Whole-Wheat Pancakes

Servings: 4

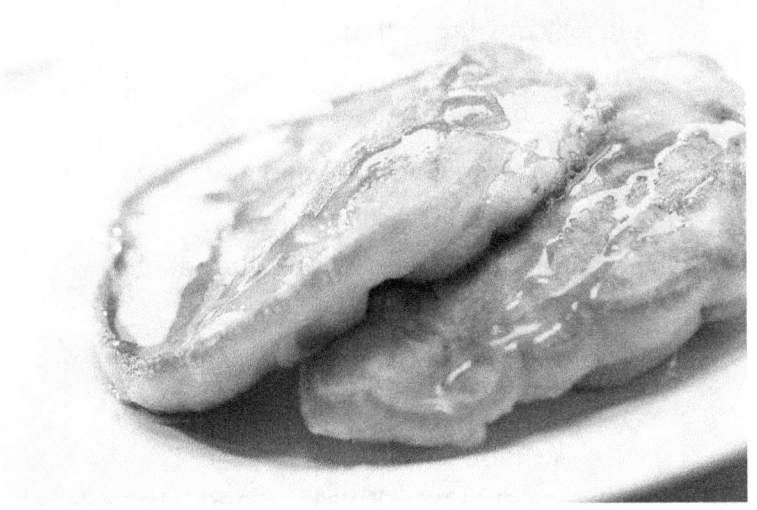

Ingredients:

- 2 cups skim milk
- 2 tablespoons apple cider vinegar
- 5 egg whites, beaten well
- ¼ cup unsweetened applesauce
- 2 cups whole-wheat flour
- 1 ½ tablespoons organic cane sugar
- 1 teaspoon baking powder
- ½ teaspoon baking soda

Instructions:

1. Whisk together the milk and vinegar in a small bowl – let rest 5 minutes.

2. Combine the dry ingredients in a mixing bowl and stir well.
3. In another bowl, beat the egg whites, applesauce, and milk mixture until smooth.
4. Whisk the wet ingredients into the dry until well combined.
5. Heat a large skillet over medium-high heat and grease with cooking spray.
6. Spoon the batter into the pan using about 2 tablespoons per pancake.
7. Cook for 2 minutes or until bubbles form in the surface of the batter then flip and cook for 2 minutes more.
8. Slide the pancakes onto a plate and repeat with the remaining batter.

Strawberry Kale Green Smoothie

Servings: 1

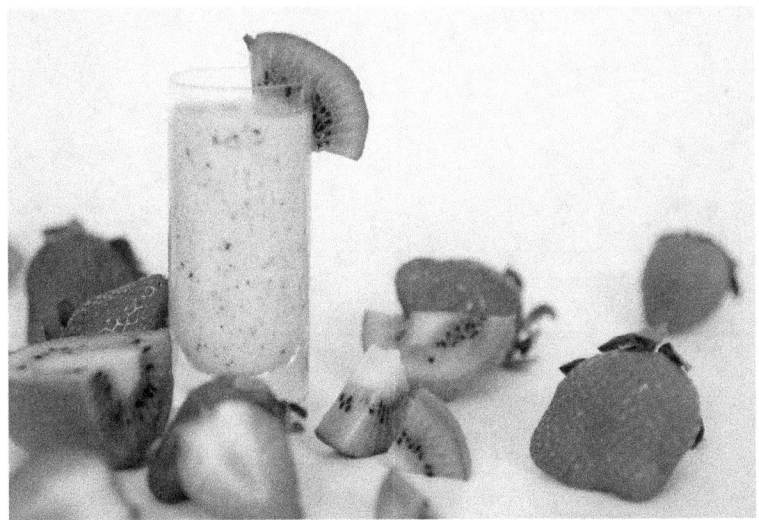

Ingredients:

- 2 cups fresh chopped kale
- ½ cup frozen sliced strawberries
- 1 ripe kiwi, peeled and sliced
- 1 cup skim milk
- ½ cup ice cubes
- 1 tablespoon ground flaxseed

Instructions:

1. Combine all of the ingredients in a high-speed blender.
2. Blend for 30 to 60 seconds on high speed until smooth.

3. Pour the smoothie into a glass and enjoy immediately.

Spinach and Mushroom Egg Cups
Servings: 12

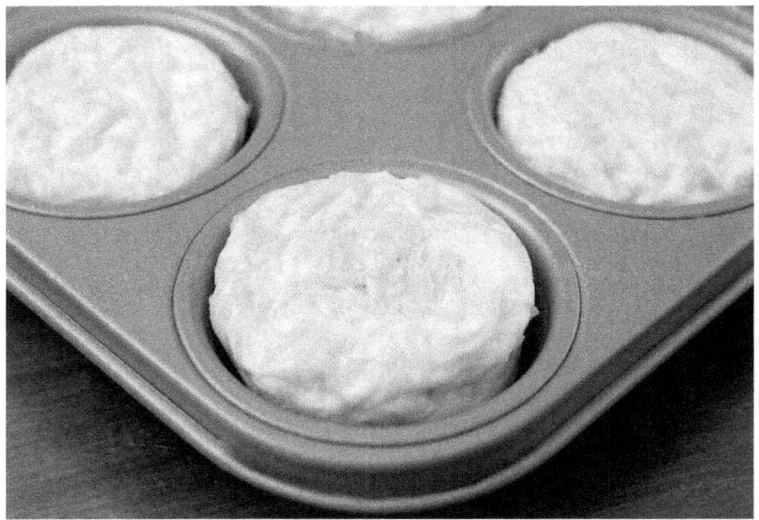

Ingredients:

- 1 cup diced mushrooms
- 1 cup diced zucchini
- 1 cup frozen spinach, thawed and moisture squeezed out
- 2 ½ cups liquid egg whites
- 3 large eggs, beaten well
- 2 tablespoons fat free milk
- Fresh ground pepper

Instructions:

1. Preheat the oven to 350°F and grease a muffin pan with cooking spray.

2. Combine the mushrooms, zucchini and spinach in a mixing bowl then spoon the mixture into the prepared muffin tin.

3. Beat together the egg whites, eggs, and milk then season with pepper.

4. Pour the egg mixture into the muffin cups, filling them almost to the top.

5. Bake for 20 to 30 minutes until the eggs are set and the tops browned.

Mixed Veggie Egg White Omelet

Servings: 1

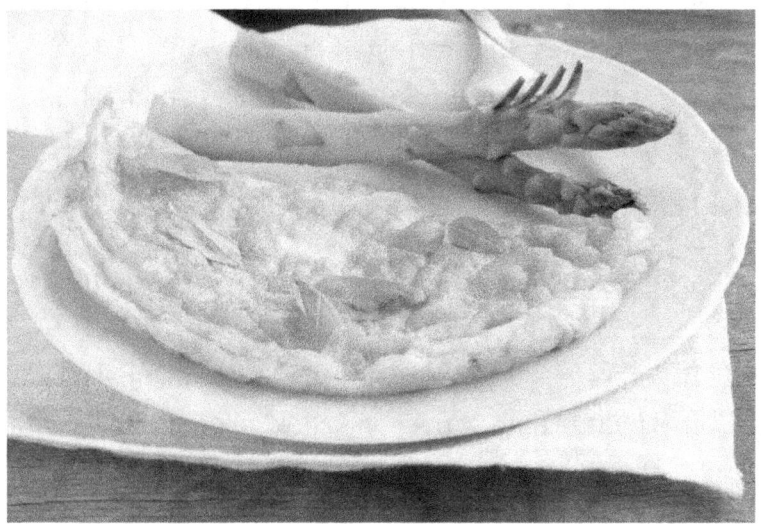

Ingredients:

- 2 teaspoons olive oil, divided
- ¼ cup fresh diced mushrooms
- ¼ cup fresh diced zucchini
- 2 tablespoons diced red pepper
- 1 clove minced garlic
- 3 large egg whites, beaten
- 1 tablespoon fresh chopped chives
- Pinch fresh ground pepper

Instructions:

1. Heat 1 teaspoon oil in a small skillet over medium heat.

2.   Add the mushrooms, red pepper, zucchini, and garlic then cook for 3 minutes.
3.   Spoon the veggie mixture into a bowl and reheat the skillet with the rest of the oil.
4.   Beat together the egg whites, chives and fresh pepper.
5.   Pour the eggs into the skillet and cook for 1 minute then stir gently.
6.   Cook the eggs for another 2 to 3 minutes until almost set.
7.   Spoon the veggie mixture over half the omelet.
8.   Fold the omelet over and cook for 1 minute or until the eggs are set.

Avocado Walnut Smoothie

Servings: 1

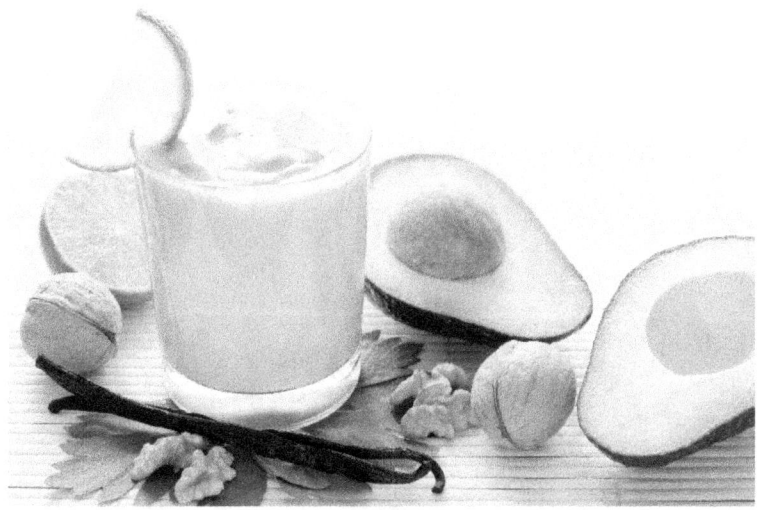

Ingredients:

- 1 small frozen banana, peeled and chopped
- ½ cup fresh chopped avocado
- 1 small stalk celery, sliced
- 2 tablespoons chopped walnuts
- 1 cup skim milk
- 1 tablespoon fresh lime juice

Instructions:

1. Combine all of the ingredients in a high-speed blender.
2. Blend for 30 to 60 seconds on high speed until smooth.

3. Pour the smoothie into a glass and enjoy immediately.

Carrot and Ginger Soup

Servings: 4 to 6

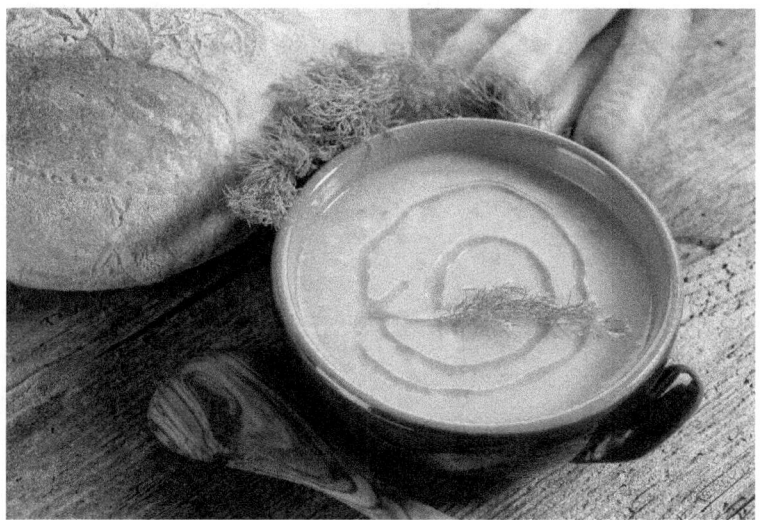

Ingredients:

- 1 tablespoon olive oil
- 1 ½ lbs. carrots, peeled and sliced
- 2 medium Yukon gold potatoes, peeled and chopped
- 1 tablespoon fresh minced ginger
- 1 tablespoon fresh minced garlic
- 6 cups vegetable broth

Instructions:

1. Heat the oil in a large saucepan over medium-high heat.
2. Add the carrots, potato, ginger and garlic and cook for 5 minutes.

3. Stir in the broth and bring the mixture to a boil.
4. Reduce heat and simmer for 25 to 30 minutes until the vegetables are tender.
5. Remove from heat and puree the soup using an immersion blender. Serve hot.

Creamy Chicken Apple Salad

Servings: 6

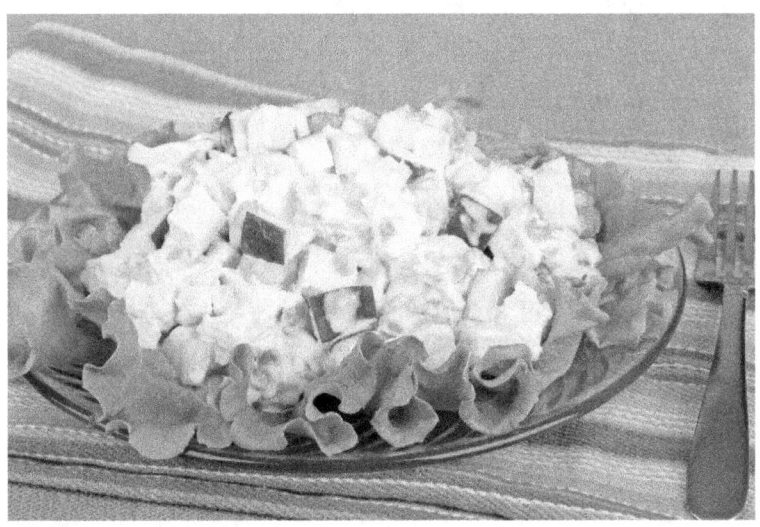

Ingredients:

- ½ cup light mayonnaise
- ½ cup fat-free yogurt, plain
- 1 tablespoon fresh lemon juice
- 1 tablespoon Dijon mustard
- 1 teaspoon raw honey
- Fresh ground pepper
- 2 lbs. boneless skinless chicken, cooked and chopped
- 1 medium ripe apple, cored and diced
- 1 large stalk celery, sliced thin
- ½ cup chopped pecans

Instructions:

1. Whisk together the mayonnaise, yogurt, lemon juice, mustard and honey in a bowl.
2. Toss in the chicken, apples, celery, and pecans to coat.
3. Season the salad with pepper and serve on a bed of fresh chopped lettuce.

Easy Tomato Basil Soup

Servings: 4 to 6

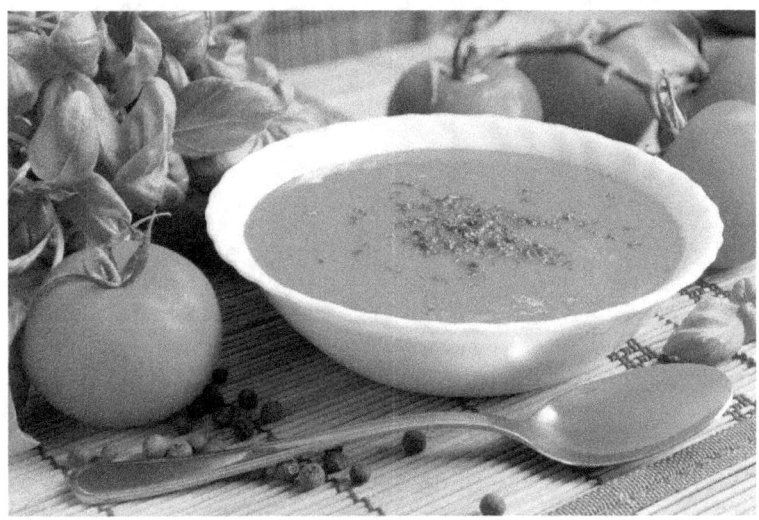

Ingredients:

1. 1 tablespoon olive oil
2. 4 (14.5-ounce) cans diced tomatoes with juice
3. 1 ½ tablespoons minced garlic
4. 5 cups vegetable or chicken broth
5. 2 ½ cups fresh chopped basil

Instructions:

1. Heat the oil in a large saucepan over medium-high heat.
2. Add the tomatoes and garlic and cook for 3 minutes.
3. Stir in the broth and bring the mixture to a boil.

4. Reduce heat and simmer for 20 to 25 minutes until the vegetables are tender.
5. Stir in the basil and cook for 2 minutes more.
6. Remove from heat and puree the soup using an immersion blender. Serve hot.

Mediterranean Chopped Salad

Servings: 4

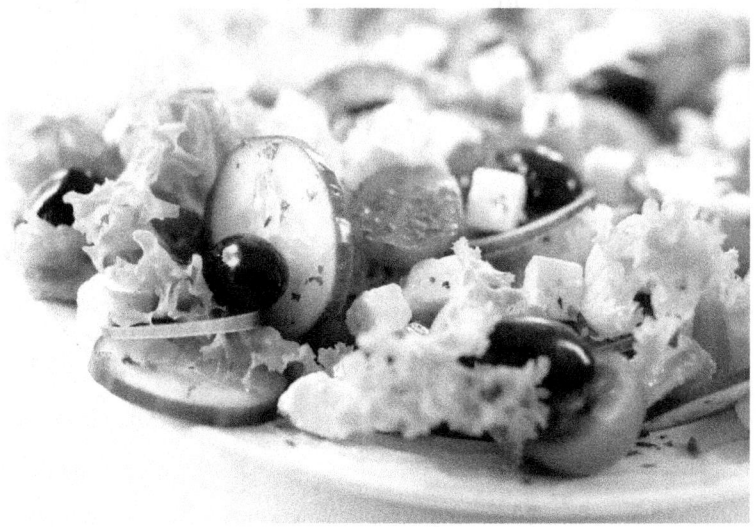

Ingredients:

- ¼ cup olive oil
- 2 tablespoons red wine vinegar
- 1 tablespoon fresh lemon juice
- 1 teaspoon assorted dried herbs (oregano, thyme, basil)
- Fresh ground pepper
- 6 cups fresh chopped lettuce
- 1 medium Roma tomato, chopped
- ½ small seedless cucumber, sliced thin
- 1 cup pitted black olives
- 1 cup low-fat feta cheese, crumbled

Instructions:

1. Whisk together the olive oil, red wine vinegar, lemon juice, herbs, and pepper in a small bowl.
2. In a salad bowl, toss together the lettuce, tomato, cucumber and olives.
3. Toss the salad with the dressing and top with feta cheese to serve.

Chicken and Vegetable Stew
Servings: 4 to 6

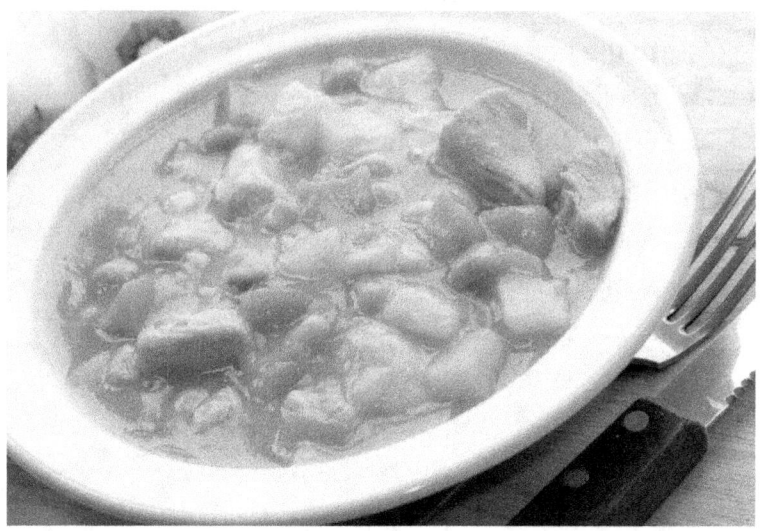

Ingredients:

- 2 tablespoons olive oil, divided
- 6 boneless skinless chicken breast halves
- Fresh ground pepper
- 4 large carrots, peeled and sliced
- 2 large Yukon gold potatoes, peeled and chopped
- 4 stalks celery, sliced
- 1 tablespoon minced garlic
- 2 tablespoons whole wheat flour
- 5 cups chicken broth
- 2 teaspoons dried tarragon
- ½ teaspoon poultry seasoning

Instructions:

1. Heat 1 tablespoon of oil in a Dutch oven over medium-high heat.
2. Season the chicken with pepper to taste and add it to the pot.
3. Cook the chicken for 5 minutes on each side until browned then transfer to a bowl.
4. Reheat the Dutch oven with the remaining oil.
5. Add the carrots, potatoes, celery and garlic then cook for 7 to 8 minutes.
6. Stir in the flour and cook for another 2 minutes.
7. Whisk in the broth and bring the mixture to a boil.
8. Chop the cooked chicken and add it to the Dutch oven along with the tarragon and poultry seasoning.
9. Reduce heat and simmer for 25 to 30 minutes until the vegetables are tender.

Dairy-Free Tuna Salad

Servings: 4 to 6

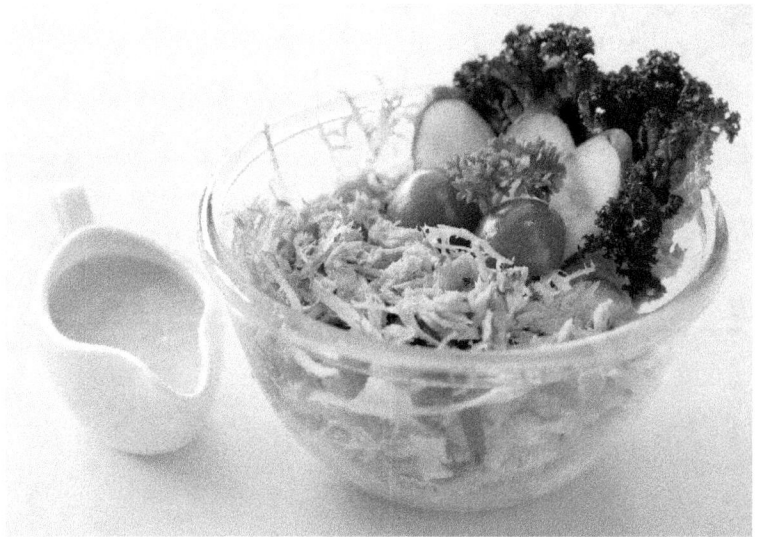

Ingredients:

- ¼ cup canned coconut milk (light)
- 1 tablespoon Dijon mustard
- 1 teaspoon lemon juice
- 3 (6-ounce) cans tuna in water, drained
- 2 stalks celery, sliced thin
- 2 green onions, sliced thin
- ¼ cup fresh chopped parsley

Instructions:

1. Whisk together the coconut milk, Dijon mustard and lemon juice in a mixing bowl.

2. Flake the tuna into the bowl and toss in the remaining ingredients.
3. Serve the salad chilled over a bed of fresh chopped lettuce.

Butternut Squash Soup with Curry

Servings: 4 to 6

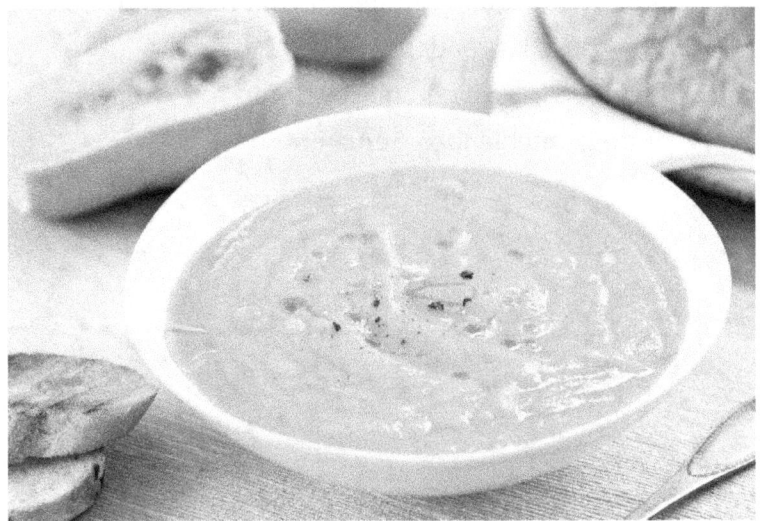

Ingredients:

- 1 tablespoon olive oil
- 2 medium carrots, peeled and chopped
- 1 stalk celery, sliced
- 4 cups fresh chopped butternut squash
- 4 cups chicken or vegetable broth
- 1 teaspoon fresh chopped thyme
- Fresh ground pepper

Instructions:

1. Heat the oil in a large saucepan over medium-high heat.
2. Add the carrots and celery then cook for 4 minutes.

3. Stir in the butternut squash, broth, thyme and pepper then bring the mixture to a boil.
4. Reduce heat and simmer for 25 to 30 minutes until the squash is tender.
5. Remove from heat and puree the soup using an immersion blender. Serve hot.

Simple Chicken Piccata

Servings: 4

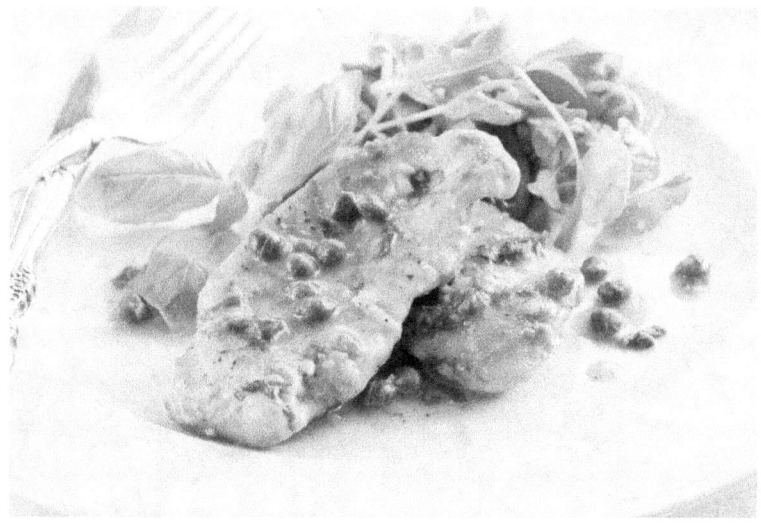

Ingredients:

- 1 lbs. boneless skinless chicken tenders
- 2 tablespoons whole-wheat flour
- ¼ cup olive oil
- 3 tablespoons fresh chopped parsley
- 2 tablespoons fresh lemon juice
- 1 tablespoon chopped capers
- Fresh ground pepper

Instructions:

1. Sandwich the chicken tenders between pieces of parchment and pound them to ¼-inch thick.
2. Toss the chicken tenders with the flour.
3. Heat the oil in a large skillet over medium-high heat.

4. Add the chicken and cook for 2 minutes on each side until evenly browned.
5. Add the parsley, lemon juice and capers and bring to a boil.
6. Reduce heat and simmer for a few minutes.
7. Season the chicken to taste with fresh ground pepper.

Grilled Balsamic Salmon Fillets

Servings: 4

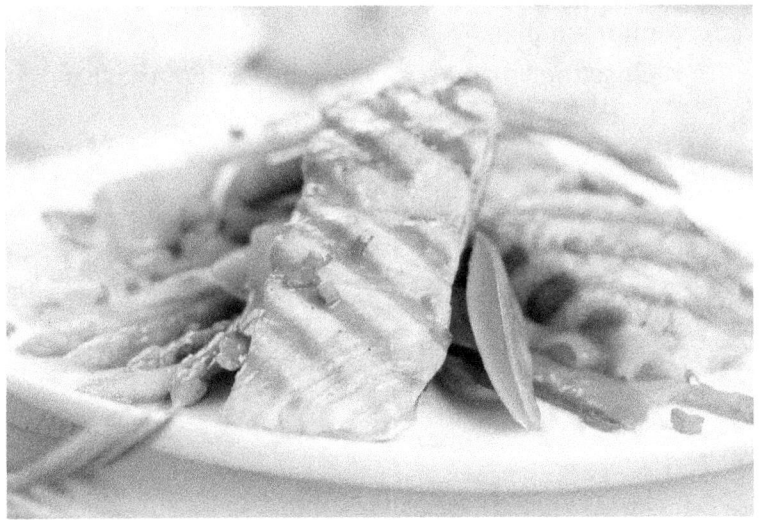

Ingredients:

- ½ cup olive oil
- ¼ cup balsamic vinegar
- 1 tablespoon Dijon mustard
- Fresh ground pepper
- 2 lbs. boneless salmon fillet

Instructions:

1. Whisk together the marinade ingredients in a bowl.
2. Cut the salmon into 2-inch chunks and place it in a shallow dish.
3. Pour the marinade over the salmon and turn to coat – let rest for 30 minutes.
4. Preheat the grill to high heat and brush the grates with oil.

5. Place the fillets on the grill upside down and cook for 2 to 3 minutes.
6. Flip the fillets and grill for 2 to 3 minutes until grill marks appear.
7. Close the lid and cook until the flesh of the fish flakes easily with a fork – don't overcook.

Turkey Meatloaf

Servings: 6 to 8

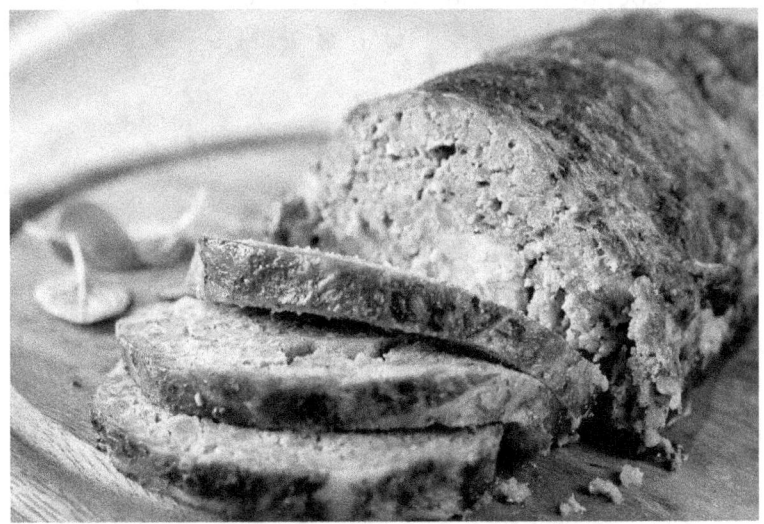

Ingredients:

- 2 lbs. lean ground turkey
- ½ cup whole-wheat breadcrumbs
- 1 small red pepper, cored and diced
- 2 large eggs, whisked well
- 1 teaspoon dried oregano
- Fresh ground pepper

Instructions:

1. Preheat the oven to 375°F.
2. Combine all of the ingredients in a mixing bowl and stir well.
3. Turn out the mixture onto a parchment-lined baking sheet and shape into a loaf.

4. Bake for 50 to 60 minutes until the meatloaf is cooked through.
5. Cool the meatloaf on a cutting board for 10 minutes before slicing to serve.

Slow Cooker Chicken Cacciatore

Servings: 6

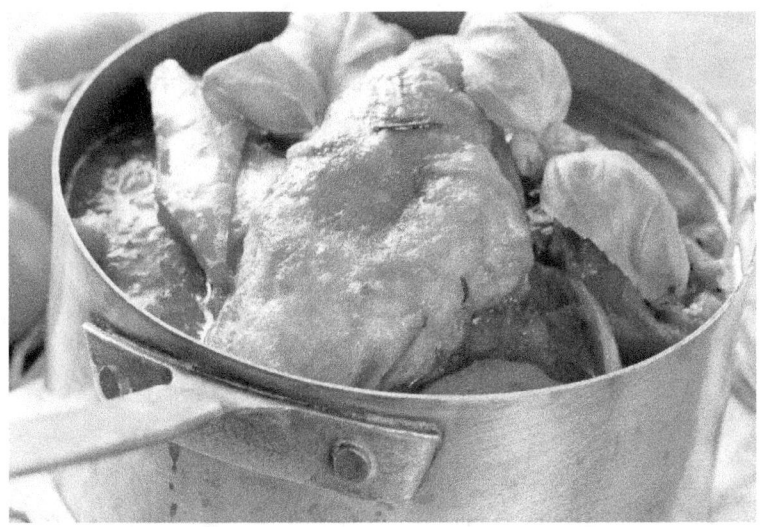

Ingredients:

- 2 tablespoons olive oil
- 3 ½ to 4 lbs. whole chicken, cut into pieces
- 1/3 cup whole-wheat flour
- 1 large red bell pepper, cored and sliced
- 1 (14.5-ounce) can diced tomatoes
- 8 ounces sliced mushrooms
- ¾ teaspoon dried oregano
- ½ teaspoon dried basil

Instructions:

1. Heat the oil in a large skillet over medium-high heat.

2. Toss the chicken with the flour and add it to the skillet – cook for 5 minutes on each side until browned.
3. Place the chicken in the bottom of the slow cooker and top with bell peppers, tomatoes, and mushrooms then sprinkle with herbs.
4. Cover the slow cooker and cook on low heat for 4 to 6 hours until the chicken is cooked through.

Almond-Crusted Baked Haddock

Servings: 4

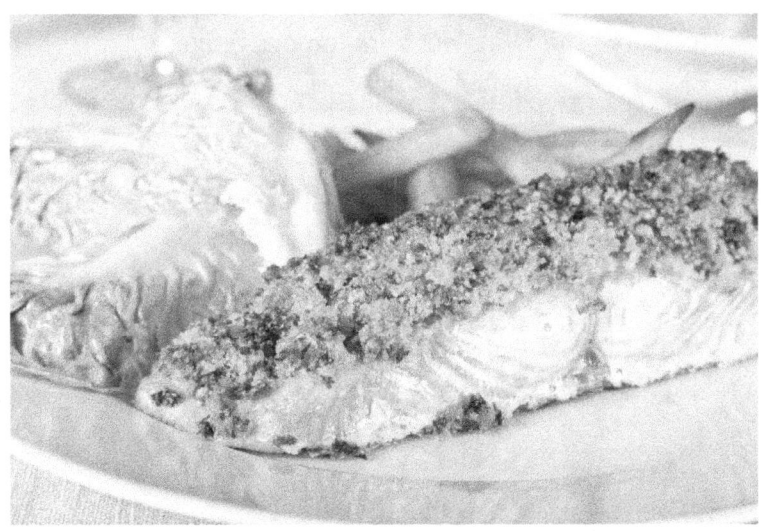

Ingredients:

- 4 (6-ounce) boneless haddock fillets
- Olive oil
- Fresh ground pepper
- ½ cup whole-wheat flour
- ¼ cup finely chopped almonds
- 1 tablespoon dried parsley

Instructions:

1. Preheat the oven to 350°F and line a baking sheet with parchment.
2. Season the fillets with pepper and brush with olive oil.
3. Combine the whole wheat flour, almonds and parsley in a mixing bowl.

4. Sprinkle the mixture over the fish in a thick layer.
5. Bake for 10 to 12 minutes until the flesh flakes easily with a fork.
6. Serve the fillets hot with lemon wedges.

Herbed Turkey Burgers

Servings: 6

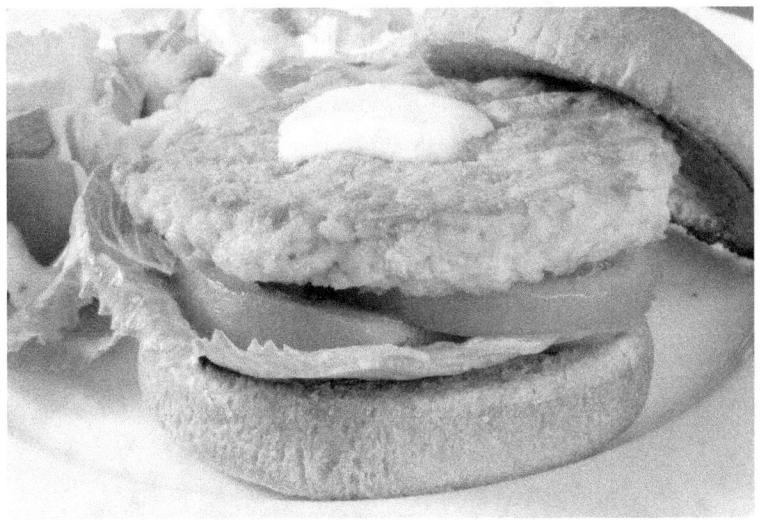

Ingredients:

- 1 lbs. lean ground turkey
- ½ cup whole-wheat breadcrumbs
- 2 tablespoons fresh chopped parsley
- 2 tablespoons fresh chopped basil
- 1 teaspoon dried oregano
- 1 tablespoon Dijon mustard
- 1 teaspoon minced garlic
- Fresh ground peppers

Instructions:

1. Preheat the broiler in your oven to high heat.
2. Combine all of the ingredients in a mixing bowl and stir well.

3. Shape the mixture by hand into 6 even-sized patties.
4. Place the patties on a broiler pan and broil for 5 minutes on each side until cooked through.
5. Serve on whole-wheat buns with your favorite burger toppings.

Baked Coconut Cod

Servings: 4

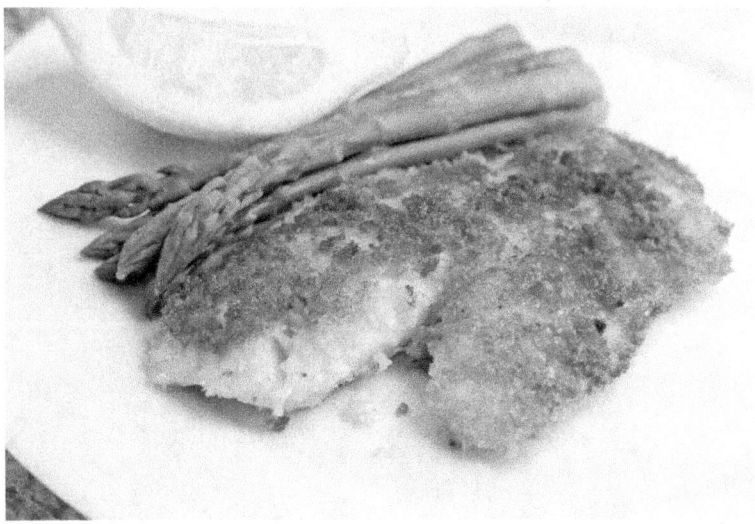

Ingredients:

- 4 (6-ounce) boneless cod fillets
- Olive oil
- Fresh ground pepper
- ¼ cup whole-wheat flour
- ½ cup unsweetened shredded coconut

Instructions:

1. Preheat the oven to 350°F and line a baking sheet with parchment.
2. Season the fillets with pepper and brush with olive oil.
3. Combine the whole wheat flour and coconut in a mixing bowl.
4. Sprinkle the mixture over the fish in a thick layer.

5. Bake for 10 to 12 minutes until the flesh flakes easily with a fork.
6. Serve the fillets hot with lemon wedges.

Chia Seed Pudding with Berries

Servings: 4

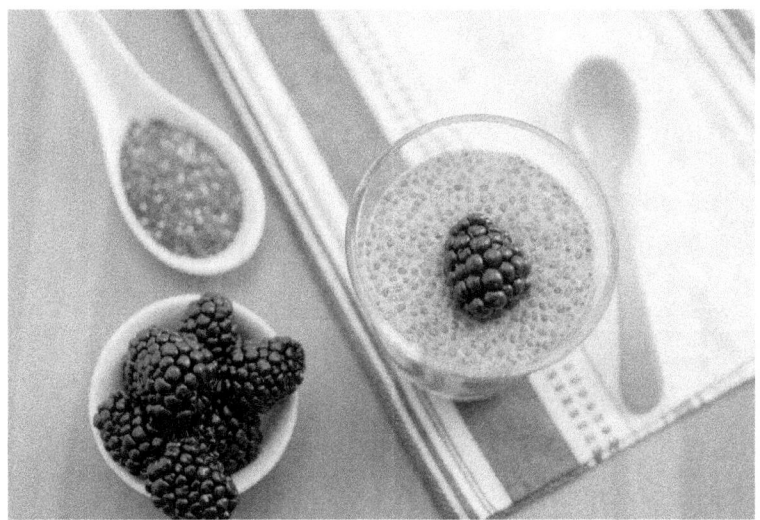

Ingredients:

- 1 cup skim milk
- 1 cup non-fat yogurt, plain
- 2 tablespoons honey
- 1 teaspoon vanilla extract
- ¼ cup chia seeds
- Fresh berries

Instructions:

1. Whisk together the milk, yogurt, honey and vanilla extract in a mixing bowl.
2. Stir in the chia seeds and let rest for 30 minutes.
3. Cover the bowl and refrigerate overnight then spoon into bowls.

4. Top the pudding with fresh berries to serve.

Honey Poached Pears

Servings: 4

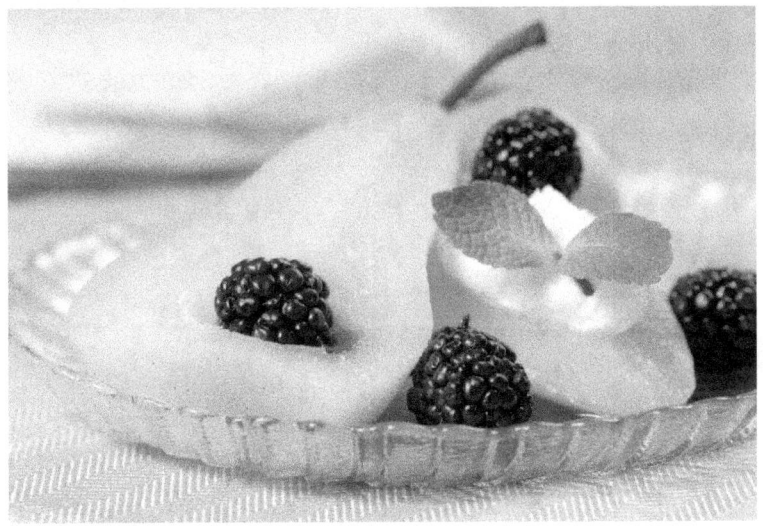

Ingredients:

- 1 cup water
- ½ cup dry white wine
- 1/3 cup raw honey
- 2 large ripe pears, peeled

Instructions:

1. Whisk together the water, wine and honey in a medium saucepan.
2. Bring the mixture to a simmer over medium heat until the honey is dissolved.
3. Cut the pears in half and remove the cores then add them to the saucepan.

4. Cover the pan and simmer on medium-low for 15 minutes until the pears are tender.
5. Remove the pears with a slotted spoon and serve drizzle with honey.

Whole-Wheat Vanilla Cupcakes

Servings: 12

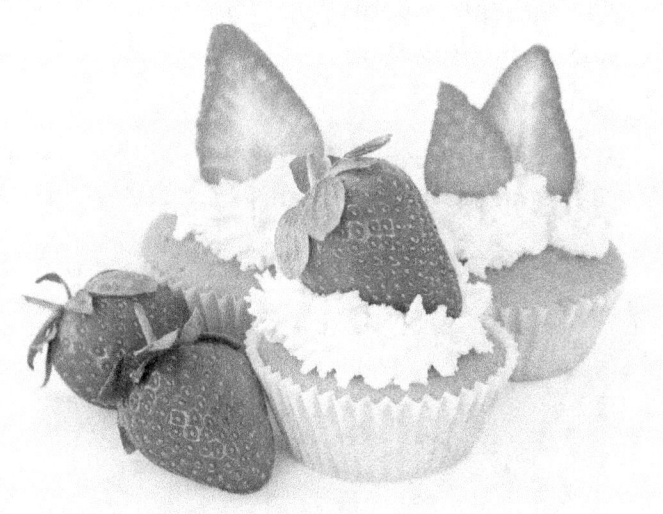

Ingredients:

- 1 ¼ cups whole-wheat white flour
- ¾ cups coconut sugar
- 1 ¼ teaspoon baking soda
- 1 cup skim milk
- 1/3 cup unsweetened applesauce
- 1 tablespoon vanilla extract
- 1 teaspoon cider vinegar

Instructions:

1. Preheat the oven to 350°F and line a muffin pan with paper liners.

2. Whisk together the flour, coconut sugar, and baking soda in a mixing bowl.
3. Stir in the milk, applesauce, vanilla extract and vinegar until smooth and lump-free.
4. Spoon the batter into the prepared pan, filling the cups ¾ full.
5. Bake for 22 to 25 minutes until a knife inserted in the center comes out clean.

Walnut-Stuffed Baked Apples

Servings: 6

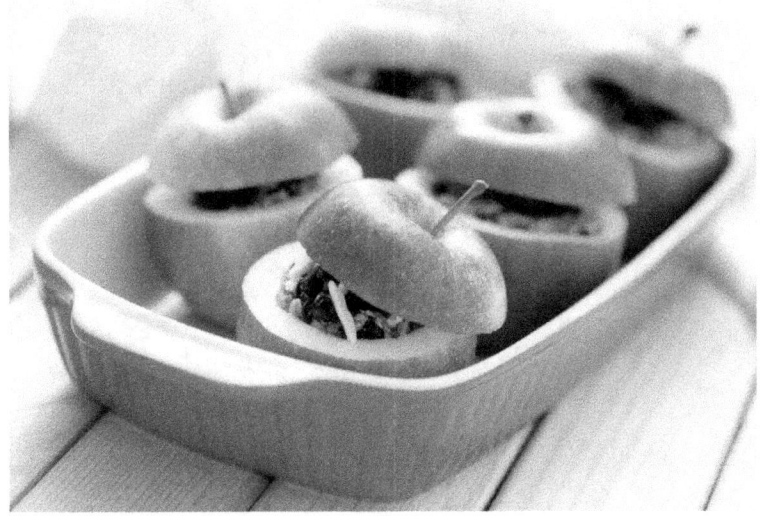

Ingredients:

- 6 medium ripe apples
- 1/3 cup coconut sugar
- 1/3 cup chopped walnuts
- 1/3 cup seedless raisins
- 1 teaspoon ground cinnamon
- 6 teaspoons grass-fed butter
- 1 cup boiling water

Instructions:

1. Preheat the oven to 375°F.
2. Slice the tops off the apples and cut out the core.
3. Combine the remaining ingredients except for the butter and boiling water in a mixing bowl.

4. Place the apples upright in a glass baking dish and spoon the filling into them.
5. Top each apple with a teaspoon of butter and pour the water into the dish.
6. Bake for 35 to 45 minutes until the apples are tender.

Cinnamon and Honey Baked Bananas

Servings: 4

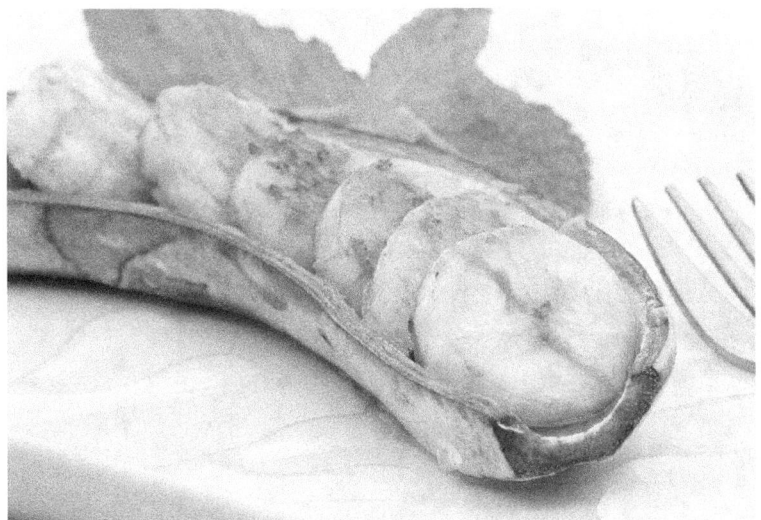

Ingredients:

- 4 large ripe bananas
- 2 tablespoons fresh lemon juice
- 2 to 3 tablespoons honey
- 1 teaspoon ground cinnamon

Instructions:

1. Preheat the oven to 400°F and grease a glass baking dish.
2. Peel the bananas and slice them in half lengthwise.
3. Place the banana halves in the baking dish and brush with lemon juice.
4. Drizzle with honey then sprinkle with cinnamon.
5. Bake the bananas for 10 to 15 minutes until tender.

Conclusion

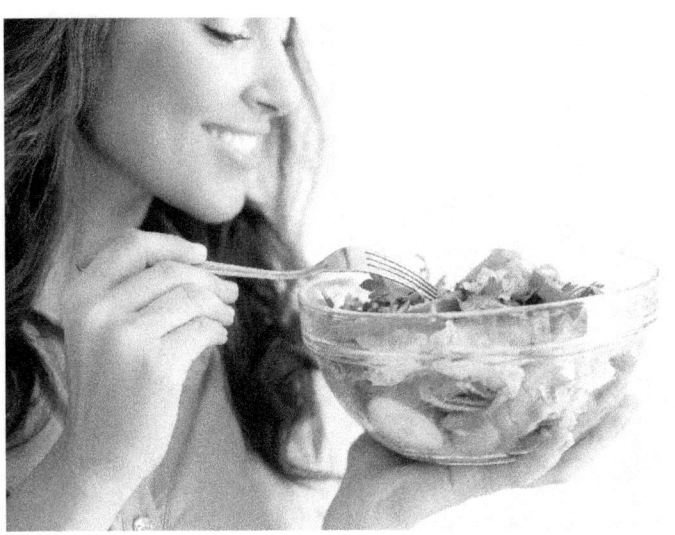

Your stubborn belly fat doesn't have to be something you resign yourself to living with forever – you can blast it away with the belly fat burner diet. This diet is not overly restrictive but you do need to be careful about how much you are eating and what you are eating. As long as you stick to four 400-calorie meals per day and eat primarily healthy fats, lean protein, fruits, vegetables, and whole grains you should be fine. If you are serious about getting rid of your stubborn belly fat, pick a recipe from this book at get started!